T0235907

MANUAL OF BIOLOGICAL MARKERS OF DISEASE